KIDNEY DISEASE FOOD CHART

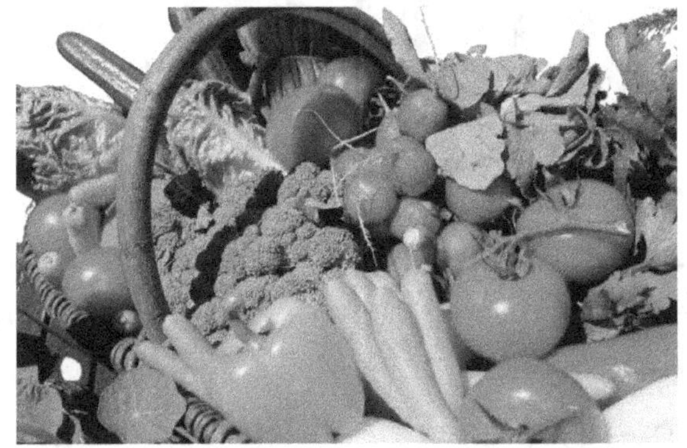

Authorized Foods for the Renal Diet - A Compilation of 300+ Low Sodium, Potassium, Phosphorus, and Protein-Rich Options Along with 30 Wholesome Recipes to Support Chronic Kidney Disease Management

Felicia O. Pace

Copyright © *Felicia O. Pace* 2024
All rights reserved. No part of this publication may be reproduced, distributed, or transmitted in any form or by any means, including photocopying, recording or other electronic or mechanical methods, without the prior written permission of the publisher, except in the case of brief quotations embodied in critical reviews and certain other non-commercial uses permitted by copyright law

For more evidence-based and approved nutrition books similar to this, explore my Amazon store. <u>HERE</u>

Table of Contents

INTRODUCTION

In a world where maintaining overall well-being is of paramount importance, understanding and managing kidney health stand out as crucial aspects of a wholesome lifestyle. Kidneys play a pivotal role in filtering and excreting waste products from the blood, regulating electrolytes, and maintaining fluid balance within the body. When the intricate balance of these functions is disrupted, it can lead to kidney diseases, imposing challenges on one's health.

The journey towards kidney health is multifaceted, encompassing medical guidance, lifestyle adjustments, and, significantly, dietary choices. Recognizing the importance of a targeted and well-balanced nutritional approach, we present the "Kidney Disease Food Chart" – a comprehensive guide with 300+ Low sodium and Low protein and 30 healthy and flavourful Recipes meticulously crafted to empower individuals on their quest for optimal kidney health.

Embarking on a journey to support kidney health can be daunting, especially with the abundance of information available. The Kidney Disease Food Chart is designed as your compass, providing clear, concise, and evidence-based guidance on what to include and avoid in your daily diet.

This book is not just a chart but a dynamic tool, carefully structured to address various aspects of kidney health, including specific nutritional values, portion control, and the avoidance of substances that may strain the kidneys. Whether you are managing chronic kidney disease, undergoing dialysis, or simply aiming for preventive care, this food chart is tailored to meet your unique dietary needs.

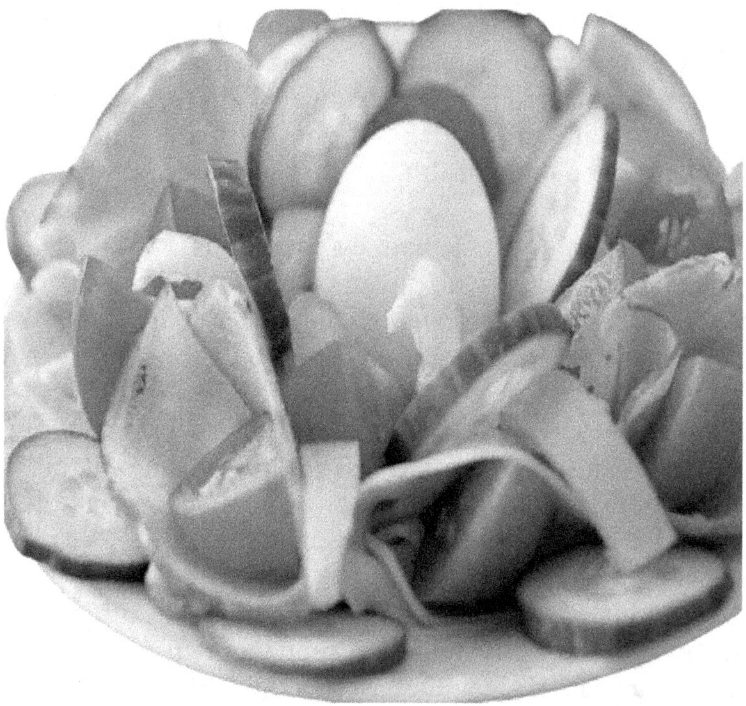

Fruits

Apples:
Calories: 95 per medium apple
Cholesterol: 0mg
Food Product Label: No added sodium, natural fruit sugars

Bananas:
Calories: 105 per medium banana
Cholesterol: 0mg
Food Product Label: No added sodium, high in potassium

Strawberries:
Calories: 4 per medium strawberry
Cholesterol: 0mg
Food Product Label: No added sodium, rich in Vitamin C

Peaches:
Calories: 60 per medium peach
Cholesterol: 0mg
Food Product Label: No added sodium, low-calorie option

Watermelon:
Calories: 46 per cup
Cholesterol: 0mg
Food Product Label: No added sodium, hydrating and low-calorie

Oranges:
Calories: 62 per medium orange
Cholesterol: 0mg
Food Product Label: No added sodium, high in Vitamin C

Grapes:
Calories: 104 per cup
Cholesterol: 0mg
Food Product Label: No added sodium, natural sugars

Kiwi:
Calories: 61 per medium kiwi
Cholesterol: 0mg
Food Product Label: No added sodium, high in dietary fiber

Pineapple:
Calories: 83 per cup
Cholesterol: 0mg
Food Product Label: No added sodium, contains bromelain enzyme

Blueberries:
Calories: 84 per cup
Cholesterol: 0mg
Food Product Label: No added sodium, rich in antioxidants

Mango:
Calories: 60 per cup
Cholesterol: 0mg
Food Product Label: No added sodium, high in Vitamin
A

Cantaloupe:
Calories: 54 per cup
Cholesterol: 0mg
Food Product Label: No added sodium, low-calorie and
hydrating

Raspberries:
Calories: 64 per cup
Cholesterol: 0mg
Food Product Label: No added sodium, high in fiber

Cranberries:
Calories: 51 per cup
Cholesterol: 0mg
Food Product Label: No added sodium, known for urinary
tract health benefits

Apricots:
Calories: 17 per apricot
Cholesterol: 0mg
Food Product Label: No added sodium, low-calorie option

Plums:
Calories: 30 per plum
Cholesterol: 0mg
Food Product Label: No added sodium, rich in Vitamin K

Pears:
Calories: 101 per medium pear
Cholesterol: 0mg
Food Product Label: No added sodium, high in dietary fiber

Cherries:
Calories: 87 per cup
Cholesterol: 0mg
Food Product Label: No added sodium, contains anthocyanins

Grapefruit:
Calories: 52 per medium grapefruit
Cholesterol: 0mg
Food Product Label: No added sodium, high in Vitamin C

Pomegranate:
Calories: 83 per cup
Cholesterol: 0mg
Food Product Label: No added sodium, rich in antioxidants

Spinach:
Calories: 7 per cup
Cholesterol: 0mg
Food Product Label: No added sodium, high in iron and vitamins

Broccoli:
Calories: 55 per cup
Cholesterol: 0mg
Food Product Label: No added sodium, rich in fiber and Vitamin C

Carrots:
Calories: 41 per cup
Cholesterol: 0mg
Food Product Label: No added sodium, excellent source of beta-carotene

Cucumbers:
Calories: 16 per cup
Cholesterol: 0mg
Food Product Label: No added sodium, hydrating and low-calorie

Bell Peppers:
Calories: 24 per cup
Cholesterol: 0mg
Food Product Label: No added sodium, high in Vitamin C

Zucchini:
Calories: 20 per cup
Cholesterol: 0mg
Food Product Label: No added sodium, low-calorie option

Tomatoes:
Calories: 32 per cup
Cholesterol: 0mg
Food Product Label: No added sodium, rich in lycopene

Cabbage:
Calories: 22 per cup
Cholesterol: 0mg
Food Product Label: No added sodium, high in fiber

Asparagus:
Calories: 27 per cup
Cholesterol: 0mg
Food Product Label: No added sodium, a good source of folate

Brussels Sprouts:
Calories: 56 per cup
Cholesterol: 0mg
Food Product Label: No added sodium, high in antioxidants

Celery:
Calories: 16 per cup
Cholesterol: 0mg
Food Product Label: No added sodium, low-calorie and crunchy

Sweet Potatoes:
Calories: 112 per medium sweet potato
Cholesterol: 0mg
Food Product Label: No added sodium, high in fiber and Vitamin A

Cauliflower:
Calories: 27 per cup
Cholesterol: 0mg
Food Product Label: No added sodium, versatile low-calorie vegetable

Green Beans:
Calories: 31 per cup
Cholesterol: 0mg
Food Product Label: No added sodium, good source of Vitamin K

Onions:
Calories: 64 per cup
Cholesterol: 0mg
Food Product Label: No added sodium, rich in antioxidants

Mushrooms:
Calories: 21 per cup
Cholesterol: 0mg
Food Product Label: No added sodium, low-calorie and rich in B-vitamins

Radishes:
Calories: 19 per cup
Cholesterol: 0mg
Food Product Label: No added sodium, crunchy and low-calorie

Eggplant:
Calories: 20 per cup
Cholesterol: 0mg
Food Product Label: No added sodium, low-calorie and versatile

Kale:
Calories: 33 per cup
Cholesterol: 0mg
Food Product Label: No added sodium, high in vitamins and minerals

Artichokes:
Calories: 60 per medium artichoke
Cholesterol: 0mg
Food Product Label: No added sodium, high in fiber and antioxidants

Lean protein

Chicken Breast:
Calories: 165 per 3.5 ounces (cooked)
Cholesterol: 73mg
Food Product Label: No added sodium, lean source of protein

Turkey Breast:
Calories: 135 per 3.5 ounces (cooked)
Cholesterol: 34mg
Food Product Label: No added sodium, low in fat and high in protein

Salmon:
Calories: 206 per 3.5 ounces (cooked)
Cholesterol: 58mg
Food Product Label: No added sodium, rich in Omega-3 fatty acids

Tofu:
Calories: 144 per 3.5 ounces (cooked)
Cholesterol: 0mg
Food Product Label: No added sodium, plant-based protein option

Shrimp:
Calories: 99 per 3.5 ounces (cooked)
Cholesterol: 189mg
Food Product Label: Low in sodium, a good source of iodine

Lean Ground Beef (90% lean):
Calories: 250 per 3.5 ounces (cooked)
Cholesterol: 86mg
Food Product Label: Limited sodium, higher protein content

Cod:
Calories: 105 per 3.5 ounces (cooked)
Cholesterol: 40mg
Food Product Label: No added sodium, low-calorie fish option

Egg Whites:
Calories: 17 per 3.5 ounces (cooked)
Cholesterol: 0mg
Food Product Label: No added sodium, low in calories and fat

Greek Yogurt (Non-fat):
Calories: 59 per 3.5 ounces
Cholesterol: 10mg
Food Product Label: Low in sodium, high in protein and probiotics

Pork Tenderloin:
Calories: 143 per 3.5 ounces (cooked)
Cholesterol: 65mg
Food Product Label: Limited sodium, lean cut of pork

Cottage Cheese (Low-fat):
Calories: 98 per 3.5 ounces
Cholesterol: 8mg
Food Product Label: Low in sodium, good source of protein and calcium

Chicken Thigh (Skinless):
Calories: 209 per 3.5 ounces (cooked)
Cholesterol: 129mg
Food Product Label: Limited sodium, higher fat content

Flank Steak:
Calories: 193 per 3.5 ounces (cooked)
Cholesterol: 62mg
Food Product Label: Limited sodium, lean beef option

Albacore Tuna:
Calories: 184 per 3.5 ounces (canned in water)
Cholesterol: 45mg
Food Product Label: No added sodium, high in protein

Lentils:
Calories: 116 per 3.5 ounces (cooked)
Cholesterol: 0mg
Food Product Label: No added sodium, plant-based protein and fiber source

Chicken Drumstick (Skinless):
Calories: 165 per 3.5 ounces (cooked)
Cholesterol: 85mg
Food Product Label: Limited sodium, dark meat option

Sardines:
Calories: 208 per 3.5 ounces (canned in water)
Cholesterol: 142mg
Food Product Label: Limited sodium, rich in Omega-3 fatty acids

Quinoa:
Calories: 120 per 3.5 ounces (cooked)
Cholesterol: 0mg
Food Product Label: No added sodium, high in protein and nutrients

Lean Ground Turkey (93% lean):
Calories: 176 per 3.5 ounces (cooked)
Cholesterol: 75mg
Food Product Label: Limited sodium, lower fat content

Halibut:
Calories: 140 per 3.5 ounces (cooked)
Cholesterol: 35mg
Food Product Label: No added sodium, lean white fish option

Whole grains

Brown Rice:
Calories: 215 per cup (cooked)
Cholesterol: 0mg
Food Product Label: No added sodium, rich in fiber and essential nutrients

Quinoa:
Calories: 222 per cup (cooked)
Cholesterol: 0mg
Food Product Label: No added sodium, complete protein source

Oats:
Calories: 154 per cup (cooked)
Cholesterol: 0mg
Food Product Label: No added sodium, high in soluble fiber

Barley:
Calories: 193 per cup (cooked)
Cholesterol: 0mg
Food Product Label: No added sodium, excellent source of fiber and vitamins

Buckwheat:
Calories: 155 per cup (cooked)
Cholesterol: 0mg
Food Product Label: No added sodium, gluten-free and high in nutrients

Millet:
Calories: 207 per cup (cooked)
Cholesterol: 0mg
Food Product Label: No added sodium, rich in antioxidants and B-vitamins

Whole Wheat Pasta:
Calories: 174 per cup (cooked)
Cholesterol: 0mg
Food Product Label: Limited sodium, higher fiber content

Farro:
Calories: 337 per cup (cooked)
Cholesterol: 0mg
Food Product Label: No added sodium, high in protein and fiber

Wild Rice:
Calories: 166 per cup (cooked)
Cholesterol: 0mg
Food Product Label: No added sodium, rich in antioxidants

Amaranth:
Calories: 251 per cup (cooked)
Cholesterol: 0mg
Food Product Label: No added sodium, gluten-free and high in protein

Whole Grain Bread:
Calories: 128 per slice
Cholesterol: 0mg
Food Product Label: Limited sodium, good source of whole grains

Brown Bread:
Calories: 82 per slice
Cholesterol: 0mg
Food Product Label: Limited sodium, high in fiber and nutrients

Bulgur:
Calories: 151 per cup (cooked)
Cholesterol: 0mg
Food Product Label: No added sodium, quick-cooking whole grain

Spelt:
Calories: 246 per cup (cooked)
Cholesterol: 0mg
Food Product Label: No added sodium, high in protein and fiber

Whole Grain Tortillas:
Calories: 96 per tortilla
Cholesterol: 0mg
Food Product Label: Limited sodium, great for wraps and sandwiches

Freekeh:
Calories: 346 per cup (cooked)
Cholesterol: 0mg
Food Product Label: No added sodium, high in fiber and protein

Sorghum:
Calories: 651 per cup (cooked)
Cholesterol: 0mg
Food Product Label: No added sodium, gluten-free whole grain

Rye:
Calories: 176 per cup (cooked)
Cholesterol: 0mg
Food Product Label: No added sodium, high in fiber and minerals

Hulled Barley:
Calories: 193 per cup (cooked)
Cholesterol: 0mg
Food Product Label: No added sodium, excellent source of fiber

Brown Basmati Rice:
Calories: 218 per cup (cooked)
Cholesterol: 0mg
Food Product Label: No added sodium, aromatic whole grain option

Legumes

Lentils:
Calories: 230 per cup (cooked)
Cholesterol: 0mg
Food Product Label: No added sodium, high in protein and fiber

Chickpeas:
Calories: 269 per cup (cooked)
Cholesterol: 0mg
Food Product Label: No added sodium, versatile and rich in nutrients

Black Beans:
Calories: 227 per cup (cooked)
Cholesterol: 0mg
Food Product Label: No added sodium, excellent source of fiber

Kidney Beans:
Calories: 225 per cup (cooked)
Cholesterol: 0mg
Food Product Label: No added sodium, high in iron and antioxidants

Cannellini Beans:
Calories: 226 per cup (cooked)
Cholesterol: 0mg
Food Product Label: No added sodium, creamy texture and rich in protein

Pinto Beans:
Calories: 245 per cup (cooked)
Cholesterol: 0mg
Food Product Label: No added sodium, good source of folate

Garbanzo Beans (Chickpeas):
Calories: 269 per cup (cooked)
Cholesterol: 0mg
Food Product Label: No added sodium, high in protein and fiber

Black-eyed Peas:
Calories: 198 per cup (cooked)
Cholesterol: 0mg
Food Product Label: No added sodium, rich in vitamins and minerals

Edamame:
Calories: 189 per cup (cooked)
Cholesterol: 0mg
Food Product Label: No added sodium, complete protein source

Lima Beans:
Calories: 209 per cup (cooked)
Cholesterol: 0mg
Food Product Label: No added sodium, high in dietary fiber

Split Peas:
Calories: 231 per cup (cooked)
Cholesterol: 0mg
Food Product Label: No added sodium, excellent source
of plant-based protein

Adzuki Beans:
Calories: 294 per cup (cooked)
Cholesterol: 0mg
Food Product Label: No added sodium, rich in
antioxidants

Butter Beans:
Calories: 209 per cup (cooked)
Cholesterol: 0mg
Food Product Label: No added sodium, creamy texture
and high in fiber

Navy Beans:
Calories: 255 per cup (cooked)
Cholesterol: 0mg
Food Product Label: No added sodium, versatile and
nutrient-dense

Red Lentils:
Calories: 230 per cup (cooked)
Cholesterol: 0mg
Food Product Label: No added sodium, quick-cooking
and high in protein

Mung Beans:
Calories: 212 per cup (cooked)
Cholesterol: 0mg
Food Product Label: No added sodium, rich in vitamins and minerals

Cranberry Beans:
Calories: 244 per cup (cooked)
Cholesterol: 0mg
Food Product Label: No added sodium, nutty flavor and high in fiber

Chana Dal (Yellow Split Peas):
Calories: 198 per cup (cooked)
Cholesterol: 0mg
Food Product Label: No added sodium, good source of protein

Great Northern Beans:
Calories: 209 per cup (cooked)
Cholesterol: 0mg
Food Product Label: No added sodium, mild flavor and high in fiber

Green Peas:
Calories: 62 per cup (cooked)
Cholesterol: 0mg
Food Product Label: No added sodium, sweet and versatile legume

Greek Yogurt (Non-fat):
Calories: 59 per 3.5 ounces
Cholesterol: 10mg
Food Product Label: Low in sodium, high in protein and probiotics

Skim Milk:
Calories: 83 per cup
Cholesterol: 5mg
Food Product Label: Low in sodium, rich in calcium and Vitamin D

Almond Milk (Unsweetened):
Calories: 13 per cup
Cholesterol: 0mg
Food Product Label: No added sodium, low in calories and a good source of Vitamin E

Cottage Cheese (Low-fat):
Calories: 98 per 3.5 ounces
Cholesterol: 8mg
Food Product Label: Low in sodium, good source of protein and calcium

String Cheese (Part-skim):
Calories: 71 per 1 ounce
Cholesterol: 15mg
Food Product Label: Low in sodium, convenient and portable snack

Plain Yogurt (Non-fat):
Calories: 137 per cup
Cholesterol: 5mg
Food Product Label: Low in sodium, versatile and can be used in various recipes

Soy Milk (Unsweetened):
Calories: 33 per cup
Cholesterol: 0mg
Food Product Label: No added sodium, plant-based alternative with protein

Ricotta Cheese (Part-skim):
Calories: 337 per cup
Cholesterol: 75mg
Food Product Label: Low in sodium, creamy texture and rich in protein

Coconut Milk (Unsweetened):
Calories: 50 per cup
Cholesterol: 0mg
Food Product Label: No added sodium, dairy-free option with a hint of coconut flavor

Low-Sodium Cheese (Various Types):
Calories: Varies based on type
Cholesterol: Varies based on type
Food Product Label: Low in sodium, suitable for those watching their salt intake

Flavored Yogurt (Low-fat):
Calories: Varies based on flavor and brand
Cholesterol: Varies based on flavor and brand
Food Product Label: Check labels for added sugars and
sodium content

Oat Milk (Unsweetened):
Calories: 80 per cup
Cholesterol: 0mg
Food Product Label: No added sodium, lactose-free
alternative

Feta Cheese (Reduced-fat):
Calories: 49 per ounce
Cholesterol: 25mg
Food Product Label: Low in sodium, adds a tangy flavor
to dishes

Swiss Cheese (Reduced-fat):
Calories: 50 per slice
Cholesterol: 26mg
Food Product Label: Low in sodium, a good source of
calcium

Cashew Milk (Unsweetened):
Calories: 25 per cup
Cholesterol: 0mg
Food Product Label: No added sodium, creamy and nutty
alternative

Mozzarella Cheese (Part-skim):
Calories: 72 per ounce
Cholesterol: 22mg
Food Product Label: Low in sodium, great for salads and pizza

Probiotic Yogurt Drinks:
Calories: Varies based on brand and serving size
Cholesterol: Varies based on brand and serving size
Food Product Label: Low in sodium, promotes gut health

Hemp Milk (Unsweetened):
Calories: 70 per cup
Cholesterol: 0mg
Food Product Label: No added sodium, plant-based and rich in omega-3 fatty acids

Low-Sodium Butter (or Margarine) Spread:
Calories: Varies based on brand and serving size
Cholesterol: Varies based on brand and serving size
Food Product Label: Low in sodium, suitable for spreading on bread or cooking

Low-Sodium Sour Cream:
Calories: Varies based on brand and serving size
Cholesterol: Varies based on brand and serving size
Food Product Label: Low in sodium, suitable for adding creaminess to dishes

Snacks

Mixed Nuts (Unsalted):
Calories: Varies based on the mix
Cholesterol: 0mg
Food Product Label: No added sodium, a source of healthy fats and protein

Air-Popped Popcorn:
Calories: 31 per cup
Cholesterol: 0mg
Food Product Label: No added sodium, high in fiber and whole grains

Rice Cakes:
Calories: 35 per rice cake
Cholesterol: 0mg
Food Product Label: Low in sodium, a light and crunchy snack

Fresh Fruit Slices:
Calories: Varies based on fruit
Cholesterol: 0mg
Food Product Label: No added sodium, natural sugars, and vitamins

Vegetable Sticks with Hummus:
Calories: Varies based on vegetables and hummus
Cholesterol: 0mg
Food Product Label: No added sodium in vegetables, check hummus label for sodium content

Seeds (e.g., Pumpkin Seeds):
Calories: Varies based on the type of seed
Cholesterol: 0mg
Food Product Label: No added sodium, rich in healthy fats
and protein

Yogurt Parfait with Berries:
Calories: Varies based on yogurt and berries
Cholesterol: Varies based on yogurt
Food Product Label: Low in sodium, high in probiotics
and antioxidants

Hard-Boiled Eggs:
Calories: 68 per large egg
Cholesterol: 186mg
Food Product Label: No added sodium, a portable and
protein-rich snack

Whole Grain Crackers:
Calories: Varies based on brand and serving size
Cholesterol: Varies based on brand and serving size
Food Product Label: Low in sodium, pair with low-
sodium cheese or hummus

Fruit Salad Cups:
Calories: Varies based on fruit
Cholesterol: 0mg
Food Product Label: No added sodium, a refreshing and
healthy snack

Dried Fruits (Unsweetened):
Calories: Varies based on the type of fruit
Cholesterol: 0mg
Food Product Label: No added sodium, a sweet and portable option

Rice Crackers:
Calories: Varies based on brand and serving size
Cholesterol: Varies based on brand and serving size
Food Product Label: Low in sodium, pair with guacamole or salsa

Low-Sodium Cheese Cubes:
Calories: Varies based on type and serving size
Cholesterol: Varies based on type
Food Product Label: Low in sodium, a convenient and protein-rich snack

Smoothie Bowl:
Calories: Varies based on ingredients
Cholesterol: Varies based on ingredients
Food Product Label: No added sodium, blend fruits and yogurt for a nutritious bowl

Hummus with Whole Grain Pita:
Calories: Varies based on hummus and pita
Cholesterol: Varies based on hummus
Food Product Label: Low in sodium, a satisfying and wholesome snack

Cucumber Slices with Cottage Cheese:
Calories: Varies based on cucumber and cottage cheese
Cholesterol: Varies based on cottage cheese
Food Product Label: Low in sodium, a refreshing and protein-packed snack

Chia Seed Pudding:
Calories: Varies based on ingredients
Cholesterol: Varies based on ingredients
Food Product Label: No added sodium, a nutritious and customizable treat

Turkey Jerky (Low-Sodium):
Calories: Varies based on brand and serving size
Cholesterol: Varies based on brand
Food Product Label: Choose low-sodium options for a protein-packed snack

Frozen Grapes:
Calories: Varies based on quantity
Cholesterol: 0mg
Food Product Label: No added sodium, a sweet and refreshing snack

Veggie Chips (Baked, Not Fried):
Calories: Varies based on brand and serving size
Cholesterol: Varies based on brand
Food Product Label: Low in sodium, choose varieties with minimal processing

Condiment and Sweeteners

Mustard:
Calories: 3 per teaspoon
Cholesterol: 0mg
Food Product Label: Low in sodium, adds flavor without extra calories

Apple Cider Vinegar:
Calories: 1 per teaspoon
Cholesterol: 0mg
Food Product Label: No added sodium, enhances taste in dressings and marinades

Balsamic Vinegar:
Calories: 14 per tablespoon
Cholesterol: 0mg
Food Product Label: Low in sodium, adds depth to salads and dishes

Lemon Juice:
Calories: 4 per tablespoon
Cholesterol: 0mg
Food Product Label: No added sodium, a refreshing and low-calorie option

Hot Sauce (Without Added Salt):
Calories: 0 per teaspoon
Cholesterol: 0mg
Food Product Label: Low in sodium, adds spice without extra calories

Soy Sauce (Low-Sodium):
Calories: 10 per tablespoon
Cholesterol: 0mg
Food Product Label: Reduced sodium option, use sparingly for flavor

Tomato Paste (No Added Salt):
Calories: 13 per 2 tablespoons
Cholesterol: 0mg
Food Product Label: Low in sodium, concentrated tomato flavor for sauces

Worcestershire Sauce (Low-Sodium):
Calories: 5 per teaspoon
Cholesterol: 0mg
Food Product Label: Reduced sodium option, adds umami to dishes

Honey:
Calories: 64 per tablespoon
Cholesterol: 0mg
Food Product Label: No added sodium, a natural sweetener with antioxidants

Maple Syrup (Pure):
Calories: 52 per tablespoon
Cholesterol: 0mg
Food Product Label: No added sodium, a natural and rich sweetener

Olive Tapenade:
Calories: Varies based on brand and serving size
Cholesterol: Varies based on brand
Food Product Label: Check labels for sodium content, a
flavorful spread

Chutney (Homemade or Low-Sodium Brands):
Calories: Varies based on ingredients and brand
Cholesterol: Varies based on ingredients and brand
Food Product Label: Opt for low-sodium options or make
your own

Salsa (Low-Sodium):
Calories: Varies based on brand and serving size
Cholesterol: Varies based on brand
Food Product Label: Choose varieties with reduced
sodium

Pesto Sauce (Homemade or Low-Sodium Brands):
Calories: Varies based on ingredients and brand
Cholesterol: Varies based on ingredients and brand
Food Product Label: Check labels for sodium content, or
make a fresh batch

Agave Nectar:
Calories: 60 per tablespoon
Cholesterol: 0mg
Food Product Label: No added sodium, a sweetener with
a lower glycemic index

Sesame Oil:
Calories: 120 per tablespoon
Cholesterol: 0mg
Food Product Label: No added sodium, imparts a rich, nutty flavor

Garlic Powder:
Calories: 9 per teaspoon
Cholesterol: 0mg
Food Product Label: No added sodium, enhances dishes without salt

Onion Powder:
Calories: 8 per teaspoon
Cholesterol: 0mg
Food Product Label: No added sodium, adds savory flavor to recipes

Cinnamon (Ground):
Calories: 6 per teaspoon
Cholesterol: 0mg
Food Product Label: No added sodium, a sweet and warm spice

Stevia (Natural Sweetener):
Calories: 0 per packet
Cholesterol: 0mg
Food Product Label: No added sodium, a calorie-free sweetener from the stevia plant

Nuts and Seeds

Almonds:
Calories: 7 per almond
Cholesterol: 0mg
Food Product Label: No added sodium, heart-healthy fats

Walnuts:
Calories: 8 per walnut half
Cholesterol: 0mg
Food Product Label: No added sodium, high in omega-3 fatty acids

Pistachios:
Calories: 4 per pistachio
Cholesterol: 0mg
Food Product Label: No added sodium, a good source of protein and fiber

Cashews:
Calories: 8 per cashew
Cholesterol: 0mg
Food Product Label: No added sodium, creamy and delicious

Brazil Nuts:
Calories: 19 per Brazil nut
Cholesterol: 0mg
Food Product Label: No added sodium, rich in selenium

Sunflower Seeds:
Calories: 5 per seed
Cholesterol: 0mg

Food Product Label: No added sodium, a crunchy and nutritious snack

Pumpkin Seeds (Pepitas):
Calories: 5 per seed
Cholesterol: 0mg
Food Product Label: No added sodium, high in iron and magnesium

Chia Seeds:
Calories: 138 per ounce
Cholesterol: 0mg
Food Product Label: No added sodium, a great source of fiber

Flaxseeds:
Calories: 37 per tablespoon
Cholesterol: 0mg
Food Product Label: No added sodium, rich in omega-3 fatty acids

Hazelnuts:
Calories: 8 per hazelnut
Cholesterol: 0mg
Food Product Label: No added sodium, a good source of vitamin E

Macadamia Nuts:
Calories: 7 per macadamia nut
Cholesterol: 0mg
Food Product Label: No added sodium, creamy and slightly sweet

Pecans:
Calories: 7 per pecan half
Cholesterol: 0mg
Food Product Label: No added sodium, rich in antioxidants

Hemp Seeds:
Calories: 166 per ounce
Cholesterol: 0mg
Food Product Label: No added sodium, a complete protein source

Sesame Seeds:
Calories: 52 per tablespoon
Cholesterol: 0mg
Food Product Label: No added sodium, adds a nutty flavor to dishes

Coconut (Shredded, Unsweetened):
Calories: 33 per tablespoon
Cholesterol: 0mg
Food Product Label: No added sodium, versatile and adds texture

Poppy Seeds:
Calories: 31 per tablespoon
Cholesterol: 0mg
Food Product Label: No added sodium, tiny seeds with a nutty flavor

Almond Butter (No Added Salt):
Calories: 98 per tablespoon
Cholesterol: 0mg
Food Product Label: No added sodium, a creamy spread

Sunflower Seed Butter (No Added Salt):
Calories: 93 per tablespoon
Cholesterol: 0mg
Food Product Label: No added sodium, a nut-free alternative

Peanuts (Dry Roasted, No Salt):
Calories: 7 per peanut
Cholesterol: 0mg
Food Product Label: No added sodium, a classic snack

Chestnuts (Roasted):
Calories: 17 per chestnut
Cholesterol: 0mg
Food Product Label: No added sodium, low in fat and a good source of vitamin C

Herbs and Spices

Basil (Dried):
Calories: 4 per tablespoon
Cholesterol: 0mg
Food Product Label: No added sodium, adds a fresh and aromatic flavor

Thyme (Dried):
Calories: 3 per teaspoon
Cholesterol: 0mg
Food Product Label: No added sodium, imparts earthy and savory notes

Oregano (Dried):
Calories: 5 per tablespoon
Cholesterol: 0mg
Food Product Label: No added sodium, a staple in Mediterranean cuisine

Rosemary (Dried):
Calories: 2 per teaspoon
Cholesterol: 0mg
Food Product Label: No added sodium, offers a piney and citrusy aroma

Cilantro (Fresh):
Calories: 0 per tablespoon
Cholesterol: 0mg
Food Product Label: No added sodium, brightens up dishes with a citrusy flavor

Parsley (Fresh):
Calories: 1 per tablespoon
Cholesterol: 0mg
Food Product Label: No added sodium, a versatile and mild herb

Chives (Fresh):
Calories: 1 per tablespoon
Cholesterol: 0mg
Food Product Label: No added sodium, adds a mild onion-like flavor

Dill (Fresh or Dried):
Calories: 3 per tablespoon (fresh), 6 per tablespoon (dried)
Cholesterol: 0mg
Food Product Label: No added sodium, complements fish and salads

Mint (Fresh):
Calories: 0 per tablespoon
Cholesterol: 0mg
Food Product Label: No added sodium, ideal for both sweet and savory dishes

Cumin (Ground):
Calories: 8 per tablespoon
Cholesterol: 0mg
Food Product Label: No added sodium, provides a warm and smoky flavor

Coriander (Ground):
Calories: 5 per tablespoon
Cholesterol: 0mg
Food Product Label: No added sodium, has a citrusy and slightly sweet taste

Paprika (Ground):
Calories: 20 per tablespoon
Cholesterol: 0mg
Food Product Label: No added sodium, adds color and a mild heat

Turmeric (Ground):
Calories: 24 per tablespoon
Cholesterol: 0mg
Food Product Label: No added sodium, known for its anti-inflammatory properties

Ginger (Ground or Fresh):
Calories: 4 per tablespoon (ground), 2 per teaspoon (fresh)
Cholesterol: 0mg
Food Product Label: No added sodium, adds warmth and depth of flavor

Cinnamon (Ground):
Calories: 6 per teaspoon
Cholesterol: 0mg
Food Product Label: No added sodium, a sweet and aromatic spice

Cloves (Ground):
Calories: 6 per teaspoon
Cholesterol: 0mg
Food Product Label: No added sodium, adds a rich and warm flavor

Cardamom (Ground):
Calories: 18 per tablespoon
Cholesterol: 0mg
Food Product Label: No added sodium, offers a sweet and spicy aroma

Fennel Seeds:
Calories: 6 per teaspoon
Cholesterol: 0mg
Food Product Label: No added sodium, has a licorice-like flavor

Sage (Dried):
Calories: 2 per teaspoon
Cholesterol: 0mg
Food Product Label: No added sodium, imparts a robust and savory taste

Allspice (Ground):
Calories: 7 per tablespoon
Cholesterol: 0mg
Food Product Label: No added sodium, combines flavors of cinnamon, cloves, and nutmeg

Olive Oil:
Calories: 119 per tablespoon
Cholesterol: 0mg
Food Product Label: No added sodium, heart-healthy monounsaturated fats

Avocado Oil:
Calories: 124 per tablespoon
Cholesterol: 0mg
Food Product Label: No added sodium, rich in monounsaturated fats and vitamin E

Coconut Oil:
Calories: 117 per tablespoon
Cholesterol: 0mg
Food Product Label: No added sodium, suitable for medium-heat cooking

Canola Oil:
Calories: 124 per tablespoon
Cholesterol: 0mg
Food Product Label: No added sodium, low in saturated fats

Flaxseed Oil:
Calories: 120 per tablespoon
Cholesterol: 0mg
Food Product Label: No added sodium, high in omega-3 fatty acids

Walnut Oil:
Calories: 120 per tablespoon
Cholesterol: 0mg
Food Product Label: No added sodium, adds a nutty flavor
to dishes

Grapeseed Oil:
Calories: 120 per tablespoon
Cholesterol: 0mg
Food Product Label: No added sodium, mild flavor and
high smoke point

Sesame Oil:
Calories: 120 per tablespoon
Cholesterol: 0mg
Food Product Label: No added sodium, imparts a rich,
nutty flavor

Sunflower Oil:
Calories: 124 per tablespoon
Cholesterol: 0mg
Food Product Label: No added sodium, versatile for
cooking and baking

Peanut Oil:
Calories: 120 per tablespoon
Cholesterol: 0mg
Food Product Label: No added sodium, suitable for high-
heat cooking

Corn Oil:
Calories: 120 per tablespoon
Cholesterol: 0mg
Food Product Label: No added sodium, a common cooking oil

Safflower Oil:
Calories: 120 per tablespoon
Cholesterol: 0mg
Food Product Label: No added sodium, ideal for frying and sautéing

Hemp Oil:
Calories: 120 per tablespoon
Cholesterol: 0mg
Food Product Label: No added sodium, a source of omega-3 and omega-6 fatty acids

Almond Oil:
Calories: 120 per tablespoon
Cholesterol: 0mg
Food Product Label: No added sodium, subtly sweet with a high smoke point

Chia Seed Oil:
Calories: 120 per tablespoon
Cholesterol: 0mg
Food Product Label: No added sodium, rich in omega-3 fatty acid

Hazelnut Oil:
Calories: 120 per tablespoon
Cholesterol: 0mg
Food Product Label: No added sodium, imparts a rich and nutty flavor

Macadamia Nut Oil:
Calories: 120 per tablespoon
Cholesterol: 0mg
Food Product Label: No added sodium, buttery and suitable for high-heat cooking

Palm Oil (Sustainably Sourced):
Calories: 120 per tablespoon
Cholesterol: 0mg
Food Product Label: No added sodium, use sparingly for its rich flavor

Rice Bran Oil:
Calories: 120 per tablespoon
Cholesterol: 0mg
Food Product Label: No added sodium, high smoke point and neutral taste

Lard (Rendered Pork Fat, Unsalted):
Calories: Varies based on type and brand
Cholesterol: Varies based on type and brand
Food Product Label: No added sodium, traditional cooking fat; choose unsalted options if available

Baking Powder (Low-Sodium):
Calories: 2 per teaspoon
Cholesterol: 0mg
Food Product Label: Reduced sodium option, leavening agent for baked goods

Baking Soda:
Calories: 0
Cholesterol: 0mg
Food Product Label: No added sodium, commonly used as a leavening agent

Vanilla Extract:
Calories: 12 per tablespoon
Cholesterol: 0mg
Food Product Label: No added sodium, enhances flavor in baking

Cocoa Powder (Unsweetened):
Calories: 12 per tablespoon
Cholesterol: 0mg
Food Product Label: No added sodium, rich chocolate flavor without added sugars

Whole Wheat Flour:
Calories: 401 per cup
Cholesterol: 0mg
Food Product Label: No added sodium, a healthier alternative to refined flour

Almond Flour:
Calories: 90 per ounce
Cholesterol: 0mg
Food Product Label: No added sodium, gluten-free option
for baking

Coconut Flour:
Calories: 60 per 1/4 cup
Cholesterol: 0mg
Food Product Label: No added sodium, absorbs moisture
and adds a subtle coconut flavor

Cornstarch:
Calories: 30 per tablespoon
Cholesterol: 0mg
Food Product Label: No added sodium, a thickening agent
for sauces and desserts

Arrowroot Powder:
Calories: 10 per tablespoon
Cholesterol: 0mg
Food Product Label: No added sodium, a natural
thickener with a neutral taste

Agar-Agar Powder:
Calories: 3 per teaspoon
Cholesterol: 0mg
Food Product Label: No added sodium, a vegetarian
alternative to gelatin

Bread Crumbs (Homemade or Low-Sodium):
Calories: Varies based on ingredients
Cholesterol: Varies based on ingredients
Food Product Label: Make your own or choose low-sodium options for coating and texture

Unsweetened Applesauce:
Calories: 49 per cup
Cholesterol: 0mg
Food Product Label: No added sodium, a natural sweetener and moisture enhancer in baking

Molasses (Unsulfured):
Calories: 58 per tablespoon
Cholesterol: 0mg
Food Product Label: No added sodium, imparts a rich, sweet flavor

Honey:
Calories: 64 per tablespoon
Cholesterol: 0mg
Food Product Label: No added sodium, a natural sweetener with antioxidants

Maple Syrup (Pure):
Calories: 52 per tablespoon
Cholesterol: 0mg
Food Product Label: No added sodium, a natural and rich sweetener

Unsweetened Coconut Flakes:
Calories: 33 per tablespoon
Cholesterol: 0mg
Food Product Label: No added sodium, adds texture and flavor to baked goods

Nutritional Yeast:
Calories: 28 per 2 tablespoons
Cholesterol: 0mg
Food Product Label: No added sodium, a savory and cheesy flavor enhancer

Xanthan Gum:
Calories: 30 per tablespoon
Cholesterol: 0mg
Food Product Label: No added sodium, gluten-free thickening agent

Ground Flaxseed:
Calories: 37 per tablespoon
Cholesterol: 0mg
Food Product Label: No added sodium, adds fiber and omega-3 fatty acids

Low-Sodium Broth (Vegetable or Chicken):
Calories: Varies based on brand and serving size
Cholesterol: Varies based on brand
Food Product Label: Choose reduced sodium options for savory recipes

Beverages

Water:
Calories: 0
Cholesterol: 0mg
Food Product Label: No added sodium, essential for hydration

Herbal Tea (Unsweetened):
Calories: 0
Cholesterol: 0mg
Food Product Label: No added sodium, a variety of flavors without caffeine

Green Tea (Unsweetened):
Calories: 0
Cholesterol: 0mg
Food Product Label: No added sodium, rich in antioxidants and mild caffeine

Black Coffee (Unsweetened):
Calories: 2 per 8-ounce cup
Cholesterol: 0mg
Food Product Label: No added sodium, a low-calorie and energizing beverage

Almond Milk (Unsweetened, Low Sodium):
Calories: 13 per cup
Cholesterol: 0mg
Food Product Label: No added sodium, a dairy-free alternative

Coconut Water:
Calories: 46 per cup
Cholesterol: 0mg
Food Product Label: Naturally low in sodium, a hydrating and electrolyte-rich option

Vegetable Juice (Low-Sodium):
Calories: Varies based on brand and serving size
Cholesterol: Varies based on brand
Food Product Label: Choose low-sodium options for a nutritious beverage

Tomato Juice (Low-Sodium):
Calories: 41 per cup
Cholesterol: 0mg
Food Product Label: Reduced sodium option, rich in vitamins and minerals

Orange Juice (Freshly Squeezed, No Added Salt):
Calories: 112 per cup
Cholesterol: 0mg
Food Product Label: No added sodium, a natural source of vitamin C

Lemonade (Homemade, Low-Sodium):
Calories: Varies based on recipe
Cholesterol: 0mg
Food Product Label: Control sodium by making your own with fresh lemons

Sparkling Water (Unflavored):
Calories: 0
Cholesterol: 0mg
Food Product Label: No added sodium, a refreshing and calorie-free option

Ginger Tea (Unsweetened):
Calories: 0
Cholesterol: 0mg
Food Product Label: No added sodium, aids digestion and has a warm flavor

Cranberry Juice (100% Pure, No Added Salt):
Calories: 116 per cup
Cholesterol: 0mg
Food Product Label: No added sodium, a tart and antioxidant-rich beverage

Chamomile Tea (Unsweetened):
Calories: 0
Cholesterol: 0mg
Food Product Label: No added sodium, promotes relaxation and good sleep

Rooibos Tea (Unsweetened):
Calories: 0
Cholesterol: 0mg
Food Product Label: No added sodium, caffeine-free with a mild and sweet taste

Pomegranate Juice (100% Pure, No Added Salt):
Calories: 134 per cup
Cholesterol: 0mg
Food Product Label: No added sodium, high in antioxidants

Iced Green Tea (Unsweetened):
Calories: 0
Cholesterol: 0mg
Food Product Label: No added sodium, a refreshing and healthy option

Mint Infused Water:
Calories: 0
Cholesterol: 0mg
Food Product Label: No added sodium, a flavorful and hydrating choice

Hibiscus Tea (Unsweetened):
Calories: 0
Cholesterol: 0mg
Food Product Label: No added sodium, vibrant in color and rich in antioxidants

Soy Milk (Unsweetened, Low Sodium):
Calories: 80 per cup
Cholesterol: 0mg
Food Product Label: No added sodium, a plant-based alternative to dairy

Vegetables

Lettuce (Iceberg):
Calories: 5 per cup
Cholesterol: 0mg
Protein: 0.5g
Food Product Label: Low in protein, great for salads

Cucumber:
Calories: 45 per cucumber
Cholesterol: 0mg
Protein: 1.9g
Food Product Label: Low in protein, refreshing and hydrating

Zucchini:
Calories: 20 per cup
Cholesterol: 0mg
Protein: 1.4g
Food Product Label: Low in protein, versatile for cooking

Spinach:
Calories: 7 per cup (cooked)
Cholesterol: 0mg
Protein: 0.9g
Food Product Label: Low in protein, high in vitamins and minerals

Bell Peppers (Green):
Calories: 19 per cup
Cholesterol: 0mg
Protein: 1.5g
Food Product Label: Low in protein, adds color and flavor

Mushrooms:
Calories: 15 per cup (sliced)
Cholesterol: 0mg
Protein: 2.2g
Food Product Label: Low in protein, a good source of vitamins

Celery:
Calories: 6 per stalk
Cholesterol: 0mg
Protein: 0.3g
Food Product Label: Low in protein, adds crunch to dishes

Cauliflower:
Calories: 27 per cup (chopped)
Cholesterol: 0mg
Protein: 2.1g
Food Product Label: Low in protein, a versatile and low-carb option

Broccoli:
Calories: 31 per cup (chopped)
Cholesterol: 0mg
Protein: 2.6g
Food Product Label: Low in protein, rich in fiber and nutrients

   KIDNEY DISEASE FOOD CHART

Asparagus:
Calories: 27 per cup
Cholesterol: 0mg
Protein: 2.9g
Food Product Label: Low in protein, a springtime favorite

Eggplant:
Calories: 20 per cup (cubed)
Cholesterol: 0mg
Protein: 0.8g
Food Product Label: Low in protein, great for roasting or grilling

Cabbage:
Calories: 22 per cup (shredded)
Cholesterol: 0mg
Protein: 1.1g
Food Product Label: Low in protein, can be used in salads or stir-fries

Brussels Sprouts:
Calories: 38 per cup (cooked)
Cholesterol: 0mg
Protein: 3.0g
Food Product Label: Low in protein, high in fiber and vitamins

Artichokes:
Calories: 60 per medium artichoke
Cholesterol: 0mg
Protein: 4.2g

Food Product Label: Low in protein, a unique addition to recipes

Radishes:
Calories: 19 per cup (sliced)
Cholesterol: 0mg
Protein: 0.8g
Food Product Label: Low in protein, adds a peppery flavor

Cress (Watercress):
Calories: 4 per cup
Cholesterol: 0mg
Protein: 0.8g
Food Product Label: Low in protein, a nutrient-dense leafy green

Turnips:
Calories: 36 per cup (cubed)
Cholesterol: 0mg
Protein: 1.2g
Food Product Label: Low in protein, a root vegetable with a mild flavor

Kale:
Calories: 33 per cup (chopped)
Cholesterol: 0mg
Protein: 2.9g
Food Product Label: Low in protein, a powerhouse of nutrients

Canned Pumpkin (Unsweetened):
Calories: 49 per cup
Cholesterol: 0mg
Protein: 2.0g
Food Product Label: Low in protein, versatile for both sweet and savory dishes

Green Beans:
Calories: 31 per cup (cooked)
Cholesterol: 0mg
Protein: 1.8g
Food Product Label: Low in protein, a classic side dish option

Fruits

Watermelon:
Calories: 46 per cup
Cholesterol: 0mg
Protein: 0.9g
Food Product Label: Low in protein, hydrating and refreshing

Strawberries:
Calories: 49 per cup (halved)
Cholesterol: 0mg
Protein: 1.0g
Food Product Label: Low in protein, high in vitamin C

Peaches:
Calories: 59 per medium peach
Cholesterol: 0mg
Protein: 1.0g

Food Product Label: Low in protein, a sweet and juicy summer fruit

Plums:
Calories: 30 per medium plum
Cholesterol: 0mg
Protein: 0.6g
Food Product Label: Low in protein, rich in antioxidants

Cantaloupe:
Calories: 60 per cup (cubed)
Cholesterol: 0mg
Protein: 1.5g
Food Product Label: Low in protein, a delicious melon option

Kiwi:
Calories: 61 per medium kiwi
Cholesterol: 0mg
Protein: 1.1g
Food Product Label: Low in protein, packed with vitamins and fiber

Blueberries:
Calories: 84 per cup
Cholesterol: 0mg
Protein: 1.1g
Food Product Label: Low in protein, high in antioxidants

Raspberries:
Calories: 65 per cup
Cholesterol: 0mg
Protein: 1.5g
Food Product Label: Low in protein, a flavorful berry option

Pineapple:
Calories: 83 per cup (chunks)
Cholesterol: 0mg
Protein: 0.9g
Food Product Label: Low in protein, tropical and sweet

Mango:
Calories: 60 per cup (sliced)
Cholesterol: 0mg
Protein: 0.8g
Food Product Label: Low in protein, a tropical delight

Grapes:
Calories: 104 per cup (red or green)
Cholesterol: 0mg
Protein: 1.1g
Food Product Label: Low in protein, a convenient and sweet snack

Oranges:
Calories: 62 per medium orange
Cholesterol: 0mg
Protein: 1.2g
Food Product Label: Low in protein, high in vitamin C

Apples:
Calories: 95 per medium apple
Cholesterol: 0mg
Protein: 0.5g
Food Product Label: Low in protein, a classic and crunchy fruit

Cherries:
Calories: 87 per cup
Cholesterol: 0mg
Protein: 1.0g
Food Product Label: Low in protein, a delicious summer treat

Apricots:
Calories: 17 per apricot (dried)
Cholesterol: 0mg
Protein: 0.5g
Food Product Label: Low in protein, a good source of fiber

Cranberries (Fresh):
Calories: 46 per cup
Cholesterol: 0mg
Protein: 0.4g
Food Product Label: Low in protein, tart and versatile

Bananas:
Calories: 105 per medium banana
Cholesterol: 0mg
Protein: 1.3g

Food Product Label: Low in protein, a convenient and potassium-rich option

Pear:
Calories: 101 per medium pear
Cholesterol: 0mg
Protein: 0.6g
Food Product Label: Low in protein, a sweet and fiber-rich fruit

Blackberries:
Calories: 62 per cup
Cholesterol: 0mg
Protein: 2.0g
Food Product Label: Low in protein, high in antioxidants

Grapefruit:
Calories: 52 per medium grapefruit
Cholesterol: 0mg
Protein: 1.0g
Food Product Label: Low in protein, a citrusy and tangy option

Grains and pseudo grains

White Rice:
Calories: 205 per cup (cooked)
Cholesterol: 0mg
Protein: 4.3g
Food Product Label: Low in protein, a staple for many cuisines

Quinoa:
Calories: 222 per cup (cooked)
Cholesterol: 0mg
Protein: 8.1g
Food Product Label: Relatively low in protein compared to other grains, a complete protein source

Couscous (Whole Wheat):
Calories: 176 per cup (cooked)
Cholesterol: 0mg
Protein: 6.0g
Food Product Label: Whole wheat couscous is lower in protein than traditional couscous

Polenta (Corn Grits):
Calories: 156 per cup (cooked)
Cholesterol: 0mg
Protein: 2.6g
Food Product Label: Low in protein, versatile for both sweet and savory dishes

Buckwheat:
Calories: 155 per cup (cooked)
Cholesterol: 0mg
Protein: 5.7g
Food Product Label: Low in protein, a gluten-free option

Barley:
Calories: 193 per cup (cooked)
Cholesterol: 0mg
Protein: 3.6g
Food Product Label: Low in protein, adds a chewy texture to dishes

Farro:
Calories: 337 per cup (cooked)
Cholesterol: 0mg
Protein: 7.3g
Food Product Label: Lower in protein compared to some other whole grains

Millet:
Calories: 207 per cup (cooked)
Cholesterol: 0mg
Protein: 6.1g
Food Product Label: Low in protein, a gluten-free option

Amaranth:
Calories: 251 per cup (cooked)
Cholesterol: 0mg
Protein: 9.3g
Food Product Label: Higher in protein for a pseudo-grain, contains all essential amino acids

White Bread (Enriched):
Calories: 79 per slice
Cholesterol: 0mg
Protein: 2.7g
Food Product Label: Low in protein, choose enriched for added nutrients

Rye Bread:
Calories: 83 per slice
Cholesterol: 0mg
Protein: 2.7g
Food Product Label: Low in protein, a hearty and flavorful option

Oats:
Calories: 154 per cup (cooked)
Cholesterol: 0mg
Protein: 5.9g
Food Product Label: Lower in protein, a versatile whole grain

White Flour (All-Purpose):
Calories: 455 per cup
Cholesterol: 0mg
Protein: 12.9g
Food Product Label: Lower protein content compared to whole grain flours

Rice Noodles:
Calories: 192 per cup (cooked)
Cholesterol: 0mg
Protein: 4.2g

Food Product Label: Low in protein, a gluten-free alternative to wheat noodles

Cornmeal:
Calories: 126 per cup
Cholesterol: 0mg
Protein: 2.2g
Food Product Label: Low in protein, used in various recipes

Sorghum:
Calories: 316 per cup (cooked)
Cholesterol: 0mg
Protein: 9.7g
Food Product Label: A gluten-free grain, relatively lower in protein

Spelt:
Calories: 246 per cup (cooked)
Cholesterol: 0mg
Protein: 10.7g
Food Product Label: A distant relative of wheat, lower in protein compared to some other grains

White Corn (Hominy):
Calories: 110 per cup (cooked)
Cholesterol: 0mg
Protein: 2.6g
Food Product Label: Lower in protein compared to other grains

White Potato:
Calories: 134 per medium potato (baked)
Cholesterol: 0mg
Protein: 3.2g
Food Product Label: Low in protein, a common and versatile starch

Cassava (Yuca):
Calories: 330 per cup (cooked)
Cholesterol: 0mg
Protein: 3.7g
Food Product Label: Low in protein, a starchy root vegetable often used in tropical cuisines

Green Beans:
Calories: 31 per cup (cooked)
Cholesterol: 0mg
Protein: 1.8g
Food Product Label: Low in protein, a classic side dish option

Snow Peas:
Calories: 26 per cup (cooked)
Cholesterol: 0mg
Protein: 2.0g
Food Product Label: Low in protein, sweet and crunchy

Snap Peas:
Calories: 41 per cup (cooked)
Cholesterol: 0mg
Protein: 2.6g
Food Product Label: Low in protein, a versatile vegetable

Lentils (Red):
Calories: 230 per cup (cooked)
Cholesterol: 0mg
Protein: 13.3g
Food Product Label: Lower in protein compared to other lentil varieties

Lima Beans:
Calories: 176 per cup (cooked)
Cholesterol: 0mg
Protein: 10.7g

Food Product Label: Lower in protein, a buttery-flavored legume

Chickpeas (Garbanzo Beans):
Calories: 269 per cup (cooked)
Cholesterol: 0mg
Protein: 14.5g
Food Product Label: Moderately low in protein, versatile for various dishes

Black-Eyed Peas:
Calories: 160 per cup (cooked)
Cholesterol: 0mg
Protein: 6.7g
Food Product Label: Lower in protein, a Southern staple

Pinto Beans:
Calories: 245 per cup (cooked)
Cholesterol: 0mg
Protein: 15.4g
Food Product Label: Lower in protein, commonly used in Mexican cuisine

Navy Beans:
Calories: 255 per cup (cooked)
Cholesterol: 0mg
Protein: 15.0g
Food Product Label: Lower in protein, often used in soups and stews

Kidney Beans:
Calories: 225 per cup (cooked)
Cholesterol: 0mg
Protein: 15.3g
Food Product Label: Lower in protein, a popular choice for chili

Cannellini Beans:
Calories: 220 per cup (cooked)
Cholesterol: 0mg
Protein: 15.4g
Food Product Label: Lower in protein, used in Italian dishes

Great Northern Beans:
Calories: 209 per cup (cooked)
Cholesterol: 0mg
Protein: 14.7g
Food Product Label: Lower in protein, similar to navy beans

Adzuki Beans:
Calories: 294 per cup (cooked)
Cholesterol: 0mg
Protein: 17.3g
Food Product Label: Lower in protein, sweet and nutty flavor

Mung Beans:
Calories: 212 per cup (cooked)
Cholesterol: 0mg
Protein: 14.2g

     KIDNEY DISEASE FOOD CHART

Food Product Label: Lower in protein, often used in Asian cuisine

Black Lentils (Beluga Lentils):
Calories: 230 per cup (cooked)
Cholesterol: 0mg
Protein: 13.3g
Food Product Label: Lower in protein, a small and flavorful lentil

Split Peas (Yellow or Green):
Calories: 231 per cup (cooked)
Cholesterol: 0mg
Protein: 16.3g
Food Product Label: Lower in protein, used in soups and stews

Fava Beans:
Calories: 187 per cup (cooked)
Cholesterol: 0mg
Protein: 13.0g
Food Product Label: Lower in protein, buttery and earthy flavor

Chana Dal (Split Chickpeas):
Calories: 160 per cup (cooked)
Cholesterol: 0mg
Protein: 8.6g
Food Product Label: Lower in protein compared to whole chickpeas

Pink Beans:
Calories: 239 per cup (cooked)
Cholesterol: 0mg
Protein: 13.0g
Food Product Label: Lower in protein, often used in Caribbean cuisine

Yellow Split Peas:
Calories: 231 per cup (cooked)
Cholesterol: 0mg
Protein: 16.3g
Food Product Label: Lower in protein, used in a variety of dishes

Dairy Alternatives

Almond Milk (Unsweetened):
Calories: 13 per cup
Cholesterol: 0mg
Protein: 1g
Food Product Label: Low in protein, a popular nut-based milk alternative

Coconut Milk (Unsweetened):
Calories: 50 per cup
Cholesterol: 0mg
Protein: 0.5g
Food Product Label: Low in protein, rich and creamy texture

Soy Milk (Unsweetened):
Calories: 80 per cup
Cholesterol: 0mg
Protein: 7g
Food Product Label: Moderately low in protein, a complete plant-based protein source

Oat Milk (Unsweetened):
Calories: 80 per cup
Cholesterol: 0mg
Protein: 3g
Food Product Label: Low in protein, known for its creamy texture

Rice Milk (Unsweetened):
Calories: 70 per cup
Cholesterol: 0mg
Protein: 0.7g
Food Product Label: Low in protein, suitable for those with allergies

Cashew Milk (Unsweetened):
Calories: 25 per cup
Cholesterol: 0mg
Protein: 0.5g
Food Product Label: Low in protein, has a mild and nutty flavor

Hemp Milk (Unsweetened):
Calories: 60 per cup
Cholesterol: 0mg
Protein: 2g
Food Product Label: Low in protein, a plant-based option with omega-3 fatty acids

Flax Milk (Unsweetened):
Calories: 25 per cup
Cholesterol: 0mg
Protein: 0.5g
Food Product Label: Low in protein, contains heart-healthy flaxseed oil

Pea Milk (Unsweetened):
Calories: 70 per cup
Cholesterol: 0mg
Protein: 8g
Food Product Label: Moderately low in protein, made from yellow peas

Hazelnut Milk (Unsweetened):
Calories: 50 per cup
Cholesterol: 0mg
Protein: 1g
Food Product Label: Low in protein, has a rich and nutty flavor

Macadamia Milk (Unsweetened):
Calories: 50 per cup
Cholesterol: 0mg
Protein: 1g
Food Product Label: Low in protein, has a creamy texture

Walnut Milk (Unsweetened):
Calories: 50 per cup
Cholesterol: 0mg
Protein: 1g
Food Product Label: Low in protein, has a distinct walnut flavor

Sunflower Seed Milk (Unsweetened):
Calories: 50 per cup
Cholesterol: 0mg
Protein: 2g
Food Product Label: Low in protein, a nut-free alternative

Ripple (Pea Protein Milk):
Calories: 70 per cup
Cholesterol: 0mg
Protein: 8g
Food Product Label: Moderately low in protein, a pea protein-based milk

Cashew Yogurt (Unsweetened):
Calories: 150 per cup
Cholesterol: 0mg
Protein: 3g
Food Product Label: Low in protein, a dairy-free yogurt alternative

Coconut Yogurt (Unsweetened):
Calories: 150 per cup
Cholesterol: 0mg
Protein: 1g
Food Product Label: Low in protein, made from coconut milk

Soy Yogurt (Unsweetened):
Calories: 150 per cup
Cholesterol: 0mg
Protein: 6g
Food Product Label: Moderately low in protein, a plant-based yogurt option

Oat Yogurt (Unsweetened):
Calories: 150 per cup
Cholesterol: 0mg
Protein: 3g
Food Product Label: Low in protein, a creamy yogurt made from oats

Almond Yogurt (Unsweetened):
Calories: 150 per cup
Cholesterol: 0mg
Protein: 5g
Food Product Label: Moderately low in protein, a dairy-free yogurt option

Rice Yogurt (Unsweetened):
Calories: 120 per cup
Cholesterol: 0mg
Protein: 1g

Food Product Label: Low in protein, a suitable option for those with allergies

Snacks

Rice Cakes:
Calories: 35 per rice cake
Cholesterol: 0mg
Protein: 0.7g
Food Product Label: Low in protein, a crunchy and versatile snack

Popcorn (Air-Popped):
Calories: 31 per cup
Cholesterol: 0mg
Protein: 1.2g
Food Product Label: Low in protein, a whole-grain snack
Vegetable Sticks (Carrots, Celery, Cucumber)

Hummus:
Calories: Varies
Cholesterol: 0mg
Protein: Varies
Food Product Label: Low in protein, a satisfying and nutritious option

Pretzels (Unsalted):
Calories: 108 per ounce
Cholesterol: 0mg
Protein: 2.6g
Food Product Label: Low in protein, a crunchy and low-fat snack

Fruit Salad:
Calories: Varies
Cholesterol: 0mg
Protein: Varies
Food Product Label: Low in protein, a sweet and refreshing snack

Seaweed Snacks:
Calories: 10 per sheet
Cholesterol: 0mg
Protein: 0.5g
Food Product Label: Low in protein, a light and crispy option

Dried Fruit Mix (Apricots, Cranberries, Raisins):
Calories: Varies
Cholesterol: 0mg
Protein: Varies
Food Product Label: Low in protein, a sweet and portable snack

Rice Crackers:
Calories: 102 per ounce
Cholesterol: 0mg
Protein: 1.2g
Food Product Label: Low in protein, available in various flavors

Vegetable Chips (Sweet Potato, Beet, Parsnip):
Calories: Varies
Cholesterol: 0mg
Protein: Varies

Food Product Label: Low in protein, a colorful and crunchy alternative

Gelatin (Sugar-Free):
Calories: 9 per tablespoon
Cholesterol: 0mg
Protein: 1.5g
Food Product Label: Low in protein, a light and sweet treat

Applesauce (Unsweetened):
Calories: 50 per cup
Cholesterol: 0mg
Protein: 0.2g
Food Product Label: Low in protein, a healthy and portable option

Trail Mix (Nuts and Seeds):
Calories: Varies
Cholesterol: Varies
Protein: Varies
Food Product Label: Choose a mix with lower protein nuts and seeds, portion-controlled for a snack

Granola Bars (Low Protein):
Calories: Varies
Cholesterol: Varies
Protein: Varies
Food Product Label: Choose options specifically labeled as low protein

Rice Krispies Treats:
Calories: 90 per treat
Cholesterol: 0mg
Protein: 0.5g
Food Product Label: Low in protein, a nostalgic and sweet
snack

Jello Cups (Sugar-Free):
Calories: 10 per cup
Cholesterol: 0mg
Protein: 2g
Food Product Label: Low in protein, a cool and refreshing
option

Fruit Sorbet:
Calories: Varies
Cholesterol: 0mg
Protein: Varies
Food Product Label: Low in protein, a dairy-free frozen
treat

Yogurt Parfait (Dairy-Free):
Calories: Varies
Cholesterol: 0mg
Protein: Varies
Food Product Label: Choose a dairy-free yogurt for a
lower protein option

Baked Potato Chips:
Calories: 152 per ounce
Cholesterol: 0mg
Protein: 2.2g
Food Product Label: Lower in protein compared to regular potato chips

Fruit Popsicles (Sugar-Free):
Calories: Varies
Cholesterol: 0mg
Protein: Varies
Food Product Label: Low in protein, a cool and fruity snack

Rice Noodle Cups (Instant):
Calories: Varies
Cholesterol: 0mg
Protein: Varies
Food Product Label: Choose options with lower protein seasoning packets for a quick and savory snack

Fats and Oil

Olive Oil:
Calories: 119 per tablespoon
Cholesterol: 0mg
Protein: 0g
Food Product Label: Low in protein, heart-healthy monounsaturated fats

Canola Oil:
Calories: 124 per tablespoon
Cholesterol: 0mg
Protein: 0g
Food Product Label: Low in protein, a versatile and neutral cooking oil

Avocado Oil:
Calories: 124 per tablespoon
Cholesterol: 0mg
Protein: 0g
Food Product Label: Low in protein, rich in monounsaturated fats

Coconut Oil:
Calories: 117 per tablespoon
Cholesterol: 0mg
Protein: 0g
Food Product Label: Low in protein, suitable for medium to high-heat cooking

Flaxseed Oil:
Calories: 120 per tablespoon
Cholesterol: 0mg
Protein: 0g
Food Product Label: Low in protein, a source of omega-3
fatty acids

Walnut Oil:
Calories: 120 per tablespoon
Cholesterol: 0mg
Protein: 0g
Food Product Label: Low in protein, adds a nutty flavor
to dishes

Grapeseed Oil:
Calories: 120 per tablespoon
Cholesterol: 0mg
Protein: 0g
Food Product Label: Low in protein, has a high smoke
point

Sesame Oil:
Calories: 120 per tablespoon
Cholesterol: 0mg
Protein: 0g
Food Product Label: Low in protein, imparts a rich, nutty
flavor

Sunflower Oil:
Calories: 124 per tablespoon
Cholesterol: 0mg
Protein: 0g

Food Product Label: Low in protein, a good source of vitamin E

Peanut Oil:
Calories: 119 per tablespoon
Cholesterol: 0mg
Protein: 0g
Food Product Label: Low in protein, suitable for high-heat cooking

Corn Oil:
Calories: 119 per tablespoon
Cholesterol: 0mg
Protein: 0g
Food Product Label: Low in protein, commonly used in cooking and frying

MCT Oil (Medium Chain Triglycerides):
Calories: 115 per tablespoon
Cholesterol: 0mg
Protein: 0g
Food Product Label: Low in protein, easily digestible source of energy

Hazelnut Oil:
Calories: 120 per tablespoon
Cholesterol: 0mg
Protein: 0g
Food Product Label: Low in protein, adds a hint of nuttiness to dishes

Almond Oil:
Calories: 120 per tablespoon
Cholesterol: 0mg
Protein: 0g
Food Product Label: Low in protein, a light and nutty oil

Safflower Oil:
Calories: 120 per tablespoon
Cholesterol: 0mg
Protein: 0g
Food Product Label: Low in protein, suitable for high-heat cooking

Chia Seed Oil:
Calories: 120 per tablespoon
Cholesterol: 0mg
Protein: 0g
Food Product Label: Low in protein, a plant-based source of omega-3s

Hemp Seed Oil:
Calories: 120 per tablespoon
Cholesterol: 0mg
Protein: 0g
Food Product Label: Low in protein, contains omega-3 and omega-6 fatty acids

Pumpkin Seed Oil:
Calories: 120 per tablespoon
Cholesterol: 0mg
Protein: 0g
Food Product Label: Low in protein, has a rich, nutty flavor

Grass-Fed Butter:
Calories: 102 per tablespoon
Cholesterol: 31mg
Protein: 0.1g
Food Product Label: Low in protein, a source of saturated fats

Ghee:
Calories: 112 per tablespoon
Cholesterol: 31mg
Protein: 0g
Food Product Label: Low in protein, clarified butter with a high smoke point

Chicken Breast (Skinless, Boneless):
Calories: 165 per 3.5 ounces (cooked)
Cholesterol: 73mg
Protein: 31g
Food Product Label: Low in fat and high in protein, a versatile and lean option.

Turkey Breast (Skinless, Boneless):
Calories: 135 per 3.5 ounces (cooked)
Cholesterol: 34mg
Protein: 30g
Food Product Label: Lean and high in protein, suitable for various dishes.

Cod:
Calories: 83 per 3.5 ounces (cooked)
Cholesterol: 49mg
Protein: 18g
Food Product Label: A low-fat fish option, rich in omega-3 fatty acids.

Tilapia:
Calories: 96 per 3.5 ounces (cooked)
Cholesterol: 55mg
Protein: 20g
Food Product Label: Mild-flavored and low in fat, a good source of protein.

Swordfish:
Calories: 206 per 3.5 ounces (cooked)
Cholesterol: 66mg
Protein: 21g
Food Product Label: A higher-fat fish, but still a good protein source when consumed in moderation.

Pork Tenderloin:
Calories: 143 per 3.5 ounces (cooked)
Cholesterol: 63mg
Protein: 24g
Food Product Label: Lean cut of pork, low in fat and high in protein.

Shrimp:
Calories: 99 per 3.5 ounces (cooked)
Cholesterol: 189mg
Protein: 21g
Food Product Label: Low in fat, a seafood option rich in protein.

Chicken Thigh (Skinless, Boneless):
Calories: 209 per 3.5 ounces (cooked)
Cholesterol: 109mg
Protein: 26g
Food Product Label: Dark meat option, still relatively lean compared to other cuts.

Ground Turkey (93% Lean):
Calories: 176 per 3.5 ounces (cooked)
Cholesterol: 76mg
Protein: 22g
Food Product Label: Leaner option for ground meat.

Salmon (Wild-Caught):
Calories: 206 per 3.5 ounces (cooked)
Cholesterol: 63mg
Protein: 22g
Food Product Label: Rich in omega-3 fatty acids, a heart-healthy option.

Lean Ground Beef (90% Lean):
Calories: 184 per 3.5 ounces (cooked)
Cholesterol: 77mg
Protein: 22g
Food Product Label: A leaner choice for ground beef.

Chicken Drumstick (Skinless):
Calories: 172 per 3.5 ounces (cooked)
Cholesterol: 108mg
Protein: 21g
Food Product Label: Dark meat option, still a good source of protein.

Tuna (Canned in Water):
Calories: 96 per 3.5 ounces (drained)
Cholesterol: 39mg
Protein: 21g
Food Product Label: A convenient and low-fat protein option.

Ground Chicken Breast:
Calories: 165 per 3.5 ounces (cooked)
Cholesterol: 93mg
Protein: 22g
Food Product Label: A leaner alternative to ground beef.

Haddock:
Calories: 88 per 3.5 ounces (cooked)
Cholesterol: 54mg
Protein: 18g
Food Product Label: Low in fat, a mild-flavored white fish.

Lean Veal:
Calories: 158 per 3.5 ounces (cooked)
Cholesterol: 112mg
Protein: 30g
Food Product Label: A lean option for those who enjoy veal.

Chicken Wing (Skinless):
Calories: 203 per 3.5 ounces (cooked)
Cholesterol: 89mg
Protein: 29g
Food Product Label: Dark meat option, moderate fat content.

Catfish:
Calories: 105 per 3.5 ounces (cooked)
Cholesterol: 47mg
Protein: 20g
Food Product Label: A lean and mild-tasting fish.

Trout:
Calories: 148 per 3.5 ounces (cooked)
Cholesterol: 58mg
Protein: 22g
Food Product Label: A flavorful fish option, rich in omega-3s.

Lean Lamb Chop:
Calories: 205 per 3.5 ounces (cooked)
Cholesterol: 89mg
Protein: 29g
Food Product Label: A leaner cut of lamb, high in protein.

Fish and seafoods

Cod:
Calories: 83 per 3.5 ounces (cooked)
Cholesterol: 49mg
Protein: 18g
Food Product Label: Low in fat, a white fish with a mild flavor.

Tilapia:
Calories: 96 per 3.5 ounces (cooked)
Cholesterol: 55mg
Protein: 20g
Food Product Label: Mild-flavored and low in fat, suitable for various dishes.

Swordfish:
Calories: 206 per 3.5 ounces (cooked)
Cholesterol: 66mg
Protein: 21g
Food Product Label: A higher-fat fish, still a good protein source in moderation.

Shrimp:
Calories: 99 per 3.5 ounces (cooked)
Cholesterol: 189mg
Protein: 21g
Food Product Label: Low in fat, a seafood option rich in protein.

Salmon (Wild-Caught):
Calories: 206 per 3.5 ounces (cooked)
Cholesterol: 63mg
Protein: 22g
Food Product Label: Rich in omega-3 fatty acids, a heart-healthy option.

Haddock:
Calories: 88 per 3.5 ounces (cooked)
Cholesterol: 54mg
Protein: 18g
Food Product Label: Low in fat, a mild-flavored white fish.

Tuna (Canned in Water):
Calories: 96 per 3.5 ounces (drained)
Cholesterol: 39mg
Protein: 21g
Food Product Label: A convenient and low-fat protein option.

Catfish:
Calories: 105 per 3.5 ounces (cooked)
Cholesterol: 47mg
Protein: 20g
Food Product Label: A lean and mild-tasting fish.

Trout:
Calories: 148 per 3.5 ounces (cooked)
Cholesterol: 58mg
Protein: 22g
Food Product Label: A flavorful fish option, rich in omega-3s.

Sardines (Canned in Water):
Calories: 208 per 3.5 ounces (drained)
Cholesterol: 142mg
Protein: 25g
Food Product Label: A small, fatty fish with high omega-3 content.

Mackerel (Atlantic):
Calories: 305 per 3.5 ounces (cooked)
Cholesterol: 105mg
Protein: 20g

Food Product Label: A fatty fish with a distinct flavor, high in omega-3s.

Scallops:
Calories: 95 per 3.5 ounces (cooked)
Cholesterol: 37mg
Protein: 20g
Food Product Label: Low in fat, a sweet and tender shellfish.

Albacore Tuna (Canned in Water):
Calories: 136 per 3.5 ounces (drained)
Cholesterol: 47mg
Protein: 29g
Food Product Label: A tuna variety with a higher protein content.

Halibut:
Calories: 140 per 3.5 ounces (cooked)
Cholesterol: 48mg
Protein: 23g
Food Product Label: A firm-textured white fish, low in fat.

Crawfish (Crayfish):
Calories: 77 per 3.5 ounces (cooked)
Cholesterol: 172mg
Protein: 14g
Food Product Label: Low in fat, a freshwater crustacean.

Clams:
Calories: 148 per 3.5 ounces (cooked)
Cholesterol: 50mg
Protein: 24g
Food Product Label: Low in fat, a shellfish with a delicate flavor.

Octopus:
Calories: 82 per 3.5 ounces (cooked)
Cholesterol: 70mg
Protein: 15g
Food Product Label: Low in fat, a unique seafood option.

Anchovies (Canned in Water):
Calories: 210 per 3.5 ounces (drained)
Cholesterol: 120mg
Protein: 29g
Food Product Label: Small, oily fish with a strong flavor.

Pollock:
Calories: 105 per 3.5 ounces (cooked)
Cholesterol: 74mg
Protein: 19g
Food Product Label: Low in fat, a mild white fish.

Mahi-Mahi:
Calories: 85 per 3.5 ounces (cooked)
Cholesterol: 58mg
Protein: 20g
Food Product Label: A lean and firm-textured fish.

Nuts and seed

Almonds:
Calories: 7 per almond
Cholesterol: 0mg
Protein: 0.3g
Food Product Label: A versatile nut, high in healthy fats.

Cashews:
Calories: 8 per cashew
Cholesterol: 0mg
Protein: 0.3g
Food Product Label: Creamy and mildly sweet, a good snack option.

Peanuts:
Calories: 4 per peanut
Cholesterol: 0mg
Protein: 0.2g
Food Product Label: A popular legume, rich in monounsaturated fats.

Walnuts:
Calories: 8 per walnut half
Cholesterol: 0mg
Protein: 0.3g
Food Product Label: High in omega-3 fatty acids, adds a nutty flavor.

Pecans:
Calories: 7 per pecan half
Cholesterol: 0mg
Protein: 0.3g

  KIDNEY DISEASE FOOD CHART

Food Product Label: Sweet and buttery, a great addition to desserts.

Hazelnuts:
Calories: 8 per hazelnut
Cholesterol: 0mg
Protein: 0.3g
Food Product Label: Nutty and versatile, suitable for various dishes.

Brazil Nuts:
Calories: 19 per Brazil nut
Cholesterol: 0mg
Protein: 0.4g
Food Product Label: High in selenium, consume in moderation.

Sunflower Seeds:
Calories: 5 per seed
Cholesterol: 0mg
Protein: 0.2g
Food Product Label: Crunchy seeds, a good source of vitamin E.

Pumpkin Seeds:
Calories: 7 per pumpkin seed
Cholesterol: 0mg
Protein: 0.3g
Food Product Label: Nutrient-dense seeds, high in zinc.

Chia Seeds:
Calories: 5 per teaspoon
Cholesterol: 0mg
Protein: 0.2g
Food Product Label: High in omega-3 fatty acids, great for thickening recipes.

Flaxseeds:
Calories: 8 per tablespoon
Cholesterol: 0mg
Protein: 0.3g
Food Product Label: Rich in fiber and omega-3 fatty acids.

Sesame Seeds:
Calories: 5 per sesame seed
Cholesterol: 0mg
Protein: 0.2g
Food Product Label: Adds a nutty flavor, rich in iron.

Macadamia Nuts:
Calories: 7 per macadamia nut
Cholesterol: 0mg
Protein: 0.3g
Food Product Label: Creamy and buttery, high in monounsaturated fats.

Chestnuts:
Calories: 17 per chestnut
Cholesterol: 0mg
Protein: 0.3g

Food Product Label: Sweet and starchy, suitable for roasting.

Hemp Seeds:
Calories: 9 per tablespoon
Cholesterol: 0mg
Protein: 1.5g
Food Product Label: Rich in omega-3s and protein.

Poppy Seeds:
Calories: 31 per tablespoon
Cholesterol: 0mg
Protein: 1g
Food Product Label: Tiny seeds, add a crunchy texture to recipes.

Almond Butter:
Calories: 98 per tablespoon
Cholesterol: 0mg
Protein: 3g
Food Product Label: A spreadable option, a good source of healthy fats.

Peanut Butter:
Calories: 94 per tablespoon
Cholesterol: 0mg
Protein: 4g
Food Product Label: Creamy or crunchy, a classic and satisfying choice.

     KIDNEY DISEASE FOOD CHART

Sunflower Seed Butter:
Calories: 94 per tablespoon
Cholesterol: 0mg
Protein: 3g
Food Product Label: Nut-free alternative, rich and creamy.

Cashew Butter:
Calories: 94 per tablespoon
Cholesterol: 0mg
Protein: 3g
Food Product Label: Smooth and slightly sweet, a delicious alternative.

Plants based protein sources

Tofu:
Calories: 94 per 3.5 ounces (raw)
Cholesterol: 0mg
Protein: 10g
Food Product Label: Versatile soy-based protein, suitable for various dishes.

Tempeh:
Calories: 195 per cup (cooked)
Cholesterol: 0mg
Protein: 21g
Food Product Label: Fermented soybean product, rich in protein and nutrients.

Edamame:
Calories: 122 per cup (cooked)
Cholesterol: 0mg
Protein: 11g
Food Product Label: Young soybeans, a tasty and protein-rich snack.

Lentils:
Calories: 230 per cup (cooked)
Cholesterol: 0mg
Protein: 18g
Food Product Label: High in fiber and protein, a versatile legume.

Chickpeas (Garbanzo Beans):
Calories: 164 per cup (cooked)
Cholesterol: 0mg
Protein: 15g
Food Product Label: A key ingredient in hummus and various dishes.

Black Beans:
Calories: 227 per cup (cooked)
Cholesterol: 0mg
Protein: 15g
Food Product Label: Rich in fiber and protein, a staple in many cuisines.

Quinoa:
Calories: 222 per cup (cooked)
Cholesterol: 0mg
Protein: 8g
Food Product Label: Complete protein source, contains all essential amino acids.

Peas:
Calories: 62 per cup (cooked)
Cholesterol: 0mg
Protein: 4g
Food Product Label: Sweet and versatile, a good source of protein.

Hemp Seeds:
Calories: 166 per ounce (shelled)
Cholesterol: 0mg
Protein: 10g
Food Product Label: Rich in omega-3s and protein.

Chia Seeds:
Calories: 138 per ounce
Cholesterol: 0mg
Protein: 5g
Food Product Label: High in fiber and omega-3 fatty acids.

Almonds:
Calories: 7 per almond
Cholesterol: 0mg
Protein: 0.3g

Food Product Label: Nutty and crunchy, a good source of healthy fats.

Peanuts:
Calories: 4 per peanut
Cholesterol: 0mg
Protein: 0.2g
Food Product Label: A popular legume, rich in monounsaturated fats.

Sunflower Seeds:
Calories: 5 per seed
Cholesterol: 0mg
Protein: 0.2g
Food Product Label: Crunchy seeds, a good source of vitamin E.

Pumpkin Seeds:
Calories: 7 per pumpkin seed
Cholesterol: 0mg
Protein: 0.3g
Food Product Label: Nutrient-dense seeds, high in zinc.

Soy Milk:
Calories: 80 per cup (unsweetened)
Cholesterol: 0mg
Protein: 8g
Food Product Label: Dairy-free milk alternative, rich in protein.

Brown Rice:
Calories: 218 per cup (cooked)
Cholesterol: 0mg
Protein: 5g
Food Product Label: A staple grain, can be used as a base in various dishes.

Spinach:
Calories: 6 per cup (cooked)
Cholesterol: 0mg
Protein: 0.9g
Food Product Label: Dark leafy green, a nutritious addition to salads and dishes.

Broccoli:
Calories: 55 per cup (cooked)
Cholesterol: 0mg
Protein: 3.7g
Food Product Label: High in fiber and protein, a cruciferous vegetable.

Seitan:
Calories: 104 per 3.5 ounces (cooked)
Cholesterol: 0mg
Protein: 21g
Food Product Label: A wheat gluten-based protein, popular in vegan diets.

Nutritional Yeast:
Calories: 60 per 2 tablespoons
Cholesterol: 0mg
Protein: 8g
Food Product Label: Adds a cheesy flavor, often used as a seasoning or in vegan dishes.

Breakfast

1. Quinoa Breakfast Bowl

Ingredients:

1/2 cup cooked quinoa

1/4 cup diced strawberries

1/4 cup blueberries

1 tablespoon chopped almonds

1 teaspoon honey

Preparation:

1. In a bowl, combine cooked quinoa, strawberries, blueberries, and chopped almonds.
2. Drizzle with honey and gently mix.
3. Serve in a bowl and enjoy!

Nutritional Information:

Calories: 250

Cholesterol: 0mg

Prep Time:

15 minutes

2. Vegetable Omelette

Ingredients:
2 large eggs
1/4 cup diced bell peppers
1/4 cup chopped spinach
1/4 cup diced tomatoes
1 tablespoon olive oil
Salt and pepper to taste

Preparation:

1. In a bowl, beat the eggs and season with salt and pepper.
2. Heat olive oil in a pan over medium heat.
3. Add bell peppers, spinach, and tomatoes to the pan and sauté until tender.
4. Pour beaten eggs over the vegetables and cook until set.
5. Fold the omelette in half and serve.

Nutritional Information:

Calories: 280
Cholesterol: 370mg

Prep Time:

20 minutes

3. Greek Yogurt Parfait

Ingredients:
1/2 cup low-fat Greek yogurt
1/4 cup granola
1/4 cup mixed berries (strawberries, blueberries, raspberries)
1 tablespoon honey

Preparation:
1. In a glass or bowl, layer Greek yogurt, granola, and mixed berries.
2. Drizzle honey on top.
3. Repeat the layers if desired.
4. Enjoy this delightful parfait!

Nutritional Information:
Calories: 300
Cholesterol: 10mg

Prep Time:
10 minutes

4. Sweet Potato and Spinach Hash

Ingredients:
1 cup diced sweet potatoes
1 cup chopped spinach
1/4 cup diced onions
1 tablespoon olive oil
1/2 teaspoon smoked paprika
Salt and pepper to taste

Preparation:
1. Heat olive oil in a skillet over medium heat.
2. Add diced sweet potatoes and cook until slightly tender.
3. Add diced onions and cook until they become translucent.
4. Stir in chopped spinach and cook until wilted.
5. Season with smoked paprika, salt, and pepper.
6. Serve hot.

Nutritional Information:
Calories: 220
Cholesterol: 0mg

Prep Time:
25 minutes

5. Berry Smoothie Bowl
Ingredients:
1/2 cup mixed berries (strawberries, blueberries, raspberries)
1/2 banana, frozen
1/2 cup low-fat yogurt
1 tablespoon chia seeds
1 tablespoon almond butter

Preparation:
1. Blend mixed berries, frozen banana, yogurt, and almond butter until smooth.
2. Pour the smoothie into a bowl.
3. Top with chia seeds and additional berries.
4. Enjoy with a spoon!

Nutritional Information:
Calories: 280
Cholesterol: 5mg

Prep Time:
10 minutes

Lunch Recipes

1. Grilled Lemon Herb Chicken with Quinoa
Ingredients:
4 oz boneless, skinless chicken breast
1 cup cooked quinoa
1 tablespoon olive oil
1 teaspoon lemon zest
1 tablespoon fresh lemon juice
1 teaspoon dried herbs (rosemary, thyme, oregano)
Salt and pepper to taste

Preparation:
1. Season chicken breast with salt, pepper, and dried herbs.
2. Grill the chicken until fully cooked.
3. In a bowl, mix cooked quinoa with olive oil, lemon zest, and lemon juice.
4. Serve the grilled chicken on a bed of lemon herb quinoa.

Nutritional Information:
Calories: 400
Cholesterol: 80mg
Prep Time:
25 minutes

2. Baked Salmon with Roasted Vegetables

Ingredients:
4 oz salmon fillet
1 cup mixed vegetables (zucchini, bell peppers, cherry tomatoes)
1 tablespoon olive oil
1 teaspoon dried dill
Salt and pepper to taste

Preparation:

1. Preheat the oven to 400°F (200°C).
2. Place salmon on a baking sheet and surround it with mixed vegetables.
3. Drizzle olive oil over the salmon and vegetables.
4. Season with dried dill, salt, and pepper.
5. Bake until salmon is cooked through and vegetables are tender.

Nutritional Information:

Calories: 350
Cholesterol: 60mg

Prep Time:

30 minutes

3. Lentil and Vegetable Stew
Ingredients:
1/2 cup dried green lentils (rinsed)
1 cup diced carrots
1 cup diced celery
1 cup diced onion
2 cloves garlic, minced
4 cups low-sodium vegetable broth
1 teaspoon dried thyme
Salt and pepper to taste

Preparation:
1. In a pot, combine lentils, carrots, celery, onion, garlic, and vegetable broth.
2. Bring to a boil, then reduce heat and simmer until lentils are tender.
3. Season with dried thyme, salt, and pepper.
4. Serve hot as a nutritious stew.

Nutritional Information:
Calories: 280
Cholesterol: 0mg

Prep Time:
40 minutes

4. Quinoa and Black Bean Salad

Ingredients:
1 cup cooked quinoa
1/2 cup black beans (canned, rinsed)
1/2 cup diced cucumber
1/2 cup cherry tomatoes, halved
2 tablespoons olive oil
1 tablespoon balsamic vinegar
1 teaspoon cumin
Salt and pepper to taste

Preparation:

1. In a bowl, combine cooked quinoa, black beans, cucumber, and cherry tomatoes.
2. In a separate bowl, whisk together olive oil, balsamic vinegar, cumin, salt, and pepper.
3. Pour the dressing over the quinoa mixture and toss to combine.
4. Chill in the refrigerator before serving.

Nutritional Information:
Calories: 320
Cholesterol: 0mg

Prep Time:
20 minutes

5. Eggplant and Tomato Stir-Fry
Ingredients:
1 cup diced eggplant
1 cup cherry tomatoes, halved
1 tablespoon olive oil
2 cloves garlic, minced
1 teaspoon dried basil
Salt and pepper to taste

Preparation:
1. Heat olive oil in a pan over medium heat.
2. Add diced eggplant and cook until slightly tender.
3. Stir in cherry tomatoes and minced garlic.
4. Season with dried basil, salt, and pepper.
5. Cook until vegetables are cooked through but still firm.

Nutritional Information:
Calories: 150
Cholesterol: 0mg

Prep Time:
15 minutes

1. Lemon Herb Baked Chicken with Roasted Vegetables
Ingredients:
4 oz boneless, skinless chicken breast
1 cup mixed vegetables (zucchini, bell peppers, cherry tomatoes)
1 tablespoon olive oil
1 teaspoon dried thyme
1 teaspoon lemon zest
Salt and pepper to taste

Preparation:
1. Preheat the oven to 400°F (200°C).
2. Season chicken breast with dried thyme, lemon zest, salt, and pepper.
3. Place the chicken on a baking sheet and surround it with mixed vegetables.
4. Drizzle olive oil over the chicken and vegetables.
5. Bake until the chicken is cooked through and vegetables are tender.

Nutritional Information:
Calories: 380
Cholesterol: 80mg

Prep Time:
30 minutes

2. Shrimp and Vegetable Stir-Fry

Ingredients:

4 oz shrimp, peeled and deveined

1 cup broccoli florets

1/2 cup sliced bell peppers

1/2 cup snap peas

2 tablespoons low-sodium soy sauce

1 tablespoon sesame oil

1 teaspoon minced ginger

1 teaspoon minced garlic

Preparation:

1. Heat sesame oil in a wok or pan over medium-high heat.
2. Add shrimp, ginger, and garlic; stir-fry until shrimp turn pink.
3. Add broccoli, bell peppers, and snap peas; continue to stir-fry until vegetables are crisp-tender.
4. Pour soy sauce over the mixture and toss until well-coated.
5. Serve hot.

Nutritional Information:

Calories: 250

Cholesterol: 150mg

Prep Time:

20 minutes

3. Baked Cod with Lemon-Dill Sauce
Ingredients:
4 oz cod fillet
1 tablespoon olive oil
1 tablespoon fresh lemon juice
1 teaspoon dried dill
1/2 teaspoon garlic powder
Salt and pepper to taste

Preparation:
1. Preheat the oven to 375°F (190°C).
2. Place cod on a baking sheet.
3. Mix olive oil, lemon juice, dried dill, garlic powder, salt, and pepper in a bowl.
4. Brush the mixture over the cod.
5. Bake until the fish is flaky and opaque.

Nutritional Information:
Calories: 180
Cholesterol: 50mg

Prep Time:
25 minutes

4. Quinoa and Vegetable Stuffed Peppers
Ingredients:
2 bell peppers, halved and seeds removed
1 cup cooked quinoa
1/2 cup black beans (canned, rinsed)
1/2 cup diced tomatoes
1/4 cup diced red onion
1/4 cup shredded low-fat cheese

1 teaspoon cumin
Salt and pepper to taste

Preparation:
1. Preheat the oven to 375°F (190°C).
2. In a bowl, combine cooked quinoa, black beans, tomatoes, red onion, cheese, cumin, salt, and pepper.
3. Stuff each bell pepper half with the quinoa mixture.
4. Place the stuffed peppers on a baking dish and bake until peppers are tender.

Nutritional Information:
Calories: 280
Cholesterol: 10mg

Prep Time:
40 minutes

5. Turkey and Vegetable Skewers
Ingredients:
4 oz turkey breast, cut into cubes
1 cup cherry tomatoes
1/2 cup red onion, cut into chunks
1/2 cup zucchini, sliced
1 tablespoon olive oil
1 teaspoon dried oregano
Salt and pepper to taste

Preparation:
1. Preheat the grill or grill pan.
2. Thread turkey, cherry tomatoes, red onion, and zucchini onto skewers.
3. In a bowl, mix olive oil, dried oregano, salt, and pepper.
4. Brush the skewers with the oil mixture.
5. Grill until the turkey is cooked through and vegetables are tender.

Nutritional Information:
Calories: 300
Cholesterol: 70mg

Prep Time:
30 minutes

Smoothies Recipes

1. Berry Blast Smoothie
Ingredients:
1/2 cup mixed berries (blueberries, strawberries, raspberries)
1/2 banana, frozen
1/2 cup low-fat Greek yogurt
1 tablespoon chia seeds
1 cup water or almond milk

Preparation:
1. Blend mixed berries, frozen banana, Greek yogurt, chia seeds, and water or almond milk until smooth.
2. Pour into a glass and enjoy this antioxidant-rich smoothie!

Nutritional Information:
Calories: 200
Cholesterol: 5mg

Prep Time:
10 minutes

2. Green Power Smoothie
Ingredients:
1 cup kale, stems removed
1/2 cucumber, peeled and sliced
1/2 green apple, cored
1/2 cup pineapple chunks
1 tablespoon flaxseeds
1 cup water or coconut water

Preparation:
1. Blend kale, cucumber, green apple, pineapple chunks, flaxseeds, and water or coconut water until smooth.
2. Pour into a glass and enjoy the refreshing and nutrient-packed green smoothie!

Nutritional Information:
Calories: 150
Cholesterol: 0mg

Prep Time:
10 minutes

3. Creamy Avocado Delight
Ingredients:
1/2 avocado, peeled and pitted
1/2 cup spinach leaves
1/2 cup mango chunks
1/2 cup low-fat yogurt
1 tablespoon honey
1 cup water or unsweetened almond milk

Preparation:
Blend avocado, spinach, mango chunks, yogurt, honey, and water or almond milk until creamy.
Pour into a glass and savor the rich and satisfying avocado smoothie!

Nutritional Information:
Calories: 250
Cholesterol: 5mg

Prep Time:
15 minutes

4. Tropical Turmeric Smoothie
Ingredients:
1/2 cup pineapple chunks
1/2 banana, frozen
1/2 teaspoon turmeric powder
1/2 teaspoon ginger, grated
1/2 cup low-fat coconut milk
1 cup water or pineapple juice

Preparation:

1. Blend pineapple chunks, frozen banana, turmeric powder, grated ginger, coconut milk, and water or pineapple juice until smooth.
2. Pour into a glass and enjoy the tropical and anti-inflammatory goodness!

Nutritional Information:
Calories: 220
Cholesterol: 0mg

Prep Time:
10 minutes

5. Cinnamon Apple Pie Smoothie

Ingredients:
1/2 cup diced apple, peeled and cored
1/2 teaspoon ground cinnamon
1/4 teaspoon nutmeg
1/2 cup low-fat vanilla yogurt
1 tablespoon almond butter
1 cup water or unsweetened apple juice

Preparation:

1. Blend diced apple, ground cinnamon, nutmeg, vanilla yogurt, almond butter, and water or apple juice until creamy.
2. Pour into a glass and relish the flavors of a comforting apple pie in a nutritious smoothie!

Nutritional Information:
Calories: 230
Cholesterol: 5mg

Prep Time:
15 minutes

Desserts Recipes

1. Chia Seed Pudding with Berries
Ingredients:
2 tablespoons chia seeds
1/2 cup unsweetened almond milk
1/2 teaspoon vanilla extract
1/2 cup mixed berries (blueberries, strawberries)

Preparation:
1. In a bowl, mix chia seeds, almond milk, and vanilla extract. Stir well.
2. Refrigerate for at least 2 hours or overnight until it thickens.
3. Top with mixed berries before serving.

Nutritional Information:
Calories: 150
Cholesterol: 0mg

Prep Time:
5 minutes (+ chilling time)

2. Avocado Chocolate Mousse
Ingredients:
1 ripe avocado
2 tablespoons cocoa powder
2 tablespoons honey
1/2 teaspoon vanilla extract
1/4 cup unsweetened almond milk

Preparation:
Blend avocado, cocoa powder, honey, vanilla extract, and almond milk until smooth.
Refrigerate for 1-2 hours before serving.

Nutritional Information:
Calories: 200
Cholesterol: 0mg

Prep Time:
10 minutes (+ chilling time)

3. Baked Apple with Cinnamon
Ingredients:
1 apple, cored and sliced
1/2 teaspoon ground cinnamon
1 tablespoon chopped walnuts
1 teaspoon honey

Preparation:
1. Preheat the oven to 375°F (190°C).
2. Place apple slices in a baking dish.
3. Sprinkle with ground cinnamon and chopped walnuts.

4. Drizzle with honey.
5. Bake until apples are tender.

Nutritional Information:
Calories: 120
Cholesterol: 0mg

Prep Time:
20 minutes

4. Coconut Rice Pudding
Ingredients:
1/2 cup cooked white rice
1 cup coconut milk
2 tablespoons honey
1/2 teaspoon vanilla extract
1/4 cup shredded coconut (unsweetened)

Preparation:
In a saucepan, combine cooked rice, coconut milk, honey,
and vanilla extract.
Simmer over low heat until it thickens.
Stir in shredded coconut.
Chill before serving.

Nutritional Information:
Calories: 220
Cholesterol: 0mg

Prep Time:
25 minutes

5. Peach and Almond Sorbet

Ingredients:
1 cup frozen peach slices
1/4 cup unsweetened almond milk
1 tablespoon almond butter
1 teaspoon honey

Preparation:
1. Blend frozen peach slices, almond milk, almond butter, and honey until smooth.
2. Scoop into a bowl or cone.
3. Garnish with sliced almonds if desired.

Nutritional Information:
Calories: 180
Cholesterol: 0mg

Prep Time:
5 minutes

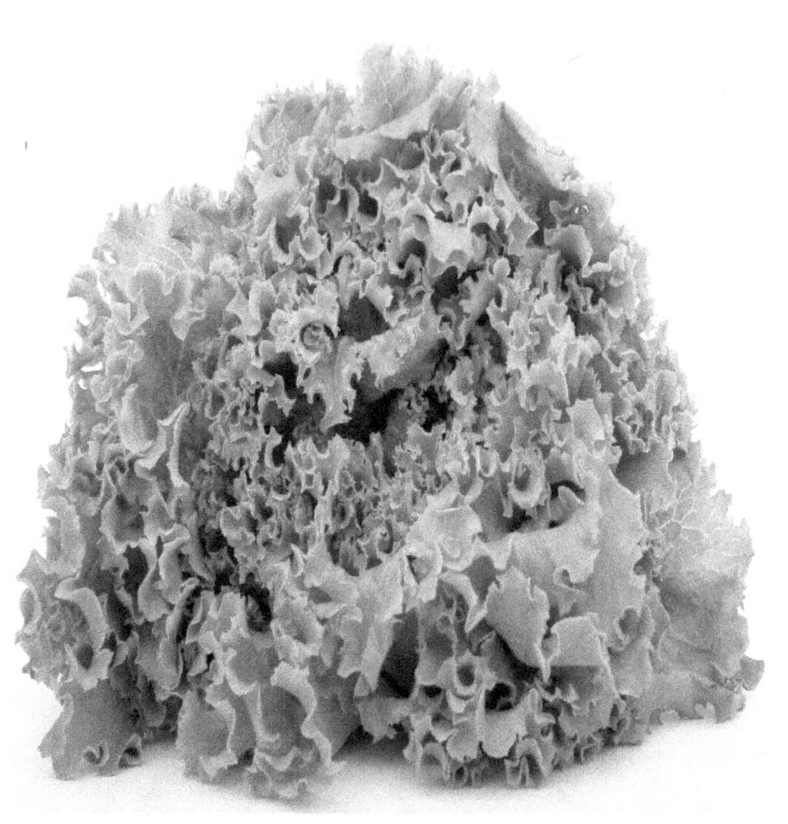

  KIDNEY DISEASE FOOD CHART

In the journey towards optimal kidney health, the Kidney Disease Food Chart stands as a beacon of guidance, offering a nuanced and practical approach to dietary choices. As we conclude this comprehensive resource, it is essential to emphasize the transformative potential it holds for individuals navigating the complexities of kidney health.

Knowledge is power, and the Kidney Disease Food Chart empowers individuals to take charge of their well-being. By providing clear insights into nutrient-rich foods, strategic meal planning, and the avoidance of renal stressors, this guide becomes a trusted ally in the pursuit of kidney wellness.

Dear Valued Readers,

I hope this book has been a source of inspiration, comfort, and valuable insights for you. Each recipe has been created with love, meticulous attention to detail, and a profound understanding of the Kidney disease foods chart ensuring heart-healthy and nutritious meals.

Your reviews, experiences, and insights hold immense value. Each evaluation motivates me to refine and customize my work to better meet your needs. Let's initiate a meaningful conversation—a dialogue that goes beyond the written words, fostering a stronger connection. Your feedback is the catalyst for ongoing improvements.

Best regards,

Felicia O. Pace

For more evidence-based and approved nutrition books similar to this, explore my Amazon store. HERE

www.ingramcontent.com/pod-product-compliance
Lightning Source LLC
Chambersburg PA
CBHW070847260726
48661CB00004B/1281